Alkaline Diet

Recipes That Are Scrumptious And Advice That Is Easy
To Follow That Will Help You Maintain A Healthy Ph
Level And Increase Your Vitality

*(These Scrumptious Foods Can Help You Lose Weight,
Improve Your Digestion, And Give You More Energy)*

Jas Belanger

TABLE OF CONTENT

What Is The Alkaline Diet?

The alkaline diet is a kind of diet that not only assists in bringing the PH level of the body back to where it should be, but also assists in keeping this level stable over the long term. All kinds of life and living creatures are dependent on certain PH levels; however, the PH values of various species are often very different from those of the human body. The meals you consume have a direct influence on the PH level in your body. The PH scale, which measures the acidity or alkalinity of the body, derives its name from the scientific term "potential of hydrogen." This is the primary reason why consuming a large quantity of food that is rich in acids may cause your body to enter a condition of acidosis, which is primarily characterised by an imbalance of the electrolytes.

This is typically lower than what your body will be based on what you consume or have eaten and the time of day; nonetheless, the human body has a range of 7.3 to 7.4 on a balanced level, with 7 being neutral; yet, the human body does have a range. It is important to take note that when the acidity levels in the body increase, the mineral levels will decrease. Therefore, you could observe a level anywhere from 5 to 7 as acidity starts to take control.

I will describe how the diet works, as well as some of the ways in which you may profit from following the diet, in the following paragraphs. There may have been shifts in the acid load of the human diet at various points in time, beginning with the time of the cave men and continuing up to the present day. The widespread industrialization of food over the course of the previous several hundred years has resulted in food crops containing greater levels of salt and decreased levels of chloride, magnesium, and potassium.

It is the job of the kidneys to keep the electrolyte levels stable, and when you eat foods that are too acidic for your body, the kidneys will utilise the electrolytes to neutralise the acid that is being produced. As a result of recent shifts in the methods through which food crops are processed, the typical American now eats three times as much salt as potassium in their diet. In addition to an increase in the amount of salt that is taken, there is also a drop in the amount of potassium, magnesium, fibre, and antioxidants. As a consequence of all of these factors, the typical diet has a significant amount of processed fats and carbohydrates.

Because of these changes, the PH level of an average person is no longer at the ideal level, and this is linked with a poor nutritional intake, particularly of magnesium and potassium. As a consequence, these changes imply that an average person's PH level is no longer at the optimal level. due of this, the effects on the body include a hastening of the ageing process, a progressive loss of organ functioning, and a lowered bone strength. This is due of the excessive acidity, which steals minerals from the bones, cells, and tissues. Additionally, this causes an increased risk of fractures.

The whole range of PH levels is 0 to 14, with 7 being considered neutral and anything over 7 being classified as basic. Anything with a PH level that is lower than 7 is considered acidic. There are a lot of individuals who try to determine their PH level by looking at their urine, and although this may be helpful as a reference, it is not completely dependable since urine is how the body flushes toxins out of the system, and this can lead to inaccurate readings of the levels. In point of fact, the best method is to place a piece of litmus paper on the tongue. It is also important to note that litmus paper can be purchased simply and at a low cost via the use of the internet. It is necessary for some areas of the body to have an acidic pH in order for the body to operate properly. An excellent illustration of this is the stomach, which is composed of acids that are responsible for digesting the food that we consume.

In the event that a person's blood falls outside of the normal PH range, this may actually be a very hazardous situation, particularly if it persists over a prolonged period of time.

The use of alkaline drinking water is a topic that might be brought up, despite the fact that it is not a fundamental component of this diet. In its most basic form, this does have a higher PH level than regular tap water, which is categorised as being somewhat acidic. It is said that the use of alkaline water provides the body with a greater number of nutrients and makes it easier to absorb those nutrients. In addition, at the current time there have not been a sufficient number of research carried out to demonstrate that drinking alkaline water does in fact result in any negative consequences on one's health. It is possible that the use of alkaline water will have a significant beneficial impact on the body, provided that the resulting alteration in PH level is consistent with what has been claimed by various persons. Although it is a very practical technique to help maintain your PH level within the normal range, it should not be relied on as the only answer. It is recommended that it be taken in moderation and in combination with a diet, with the majority of the alkalizing benefits coming from the food that you eat.

Because the foods included in this diet plan are almost entirely composed of vegetables and fruits, it is an excellent option for those who follow a vegetarian or vegan lifestyle.

The included recipes were not developed with the purpose of using meats as a major source of protein; however, one or two of the dishes do use meat or fish as the primary source of protein since they were developed as a balanced meal, giving the 80/20 split of alkalizing and other foods that is advised. If you read a recipe and it calls for meat or fish, you have two options: either leave out the meat or fish and continue with the recipe as written, or you may add anything to the dish that acts as a meat or fish alternative and it could work just as well. In any case, the decision is yours to make since they have been developed to be very customizable and diverse in flavour, so you are sure to find something there that will sate your hunger.

As is the case with the vast majority of dietary plans, it is wise to obtain the advice of a qualified medical expert before beginning the ketogenic diet, particularly if you are currently on any kind of medicine or suffer from any kind of sickness or illness. Even though it is not the primary focus of this book, one of the best pieces of advice that can be given is to complete the suggested amount of physical activity each day, which is thirty minutes. This does not have to be anything very strenuous; it may be as simple as squats or stretches that you can do in the comfort of your own home. You can break this up into two 15-minute sessions, one in the morning and one in the evening. Because your body goes through daily changes, it is crucial to remember that if you are following this diet in order to lose weight, you should limit the number of times that you weigh yourself to once or maybe twice per week. Because your body goes through daily changes, it may seem as if you have gained weight instead of losing it, but this may not be the case. Keep a cheerful attitude each and every day.

The Advantages Of Adopting An Alkaline Diet

There is always a diet that can be tailored to fit a person's preferences, regardless of the kinds of foods that they like eating the most. Because there are so many different diets available today, it may be tough to determine which one is the most effective. However, the alkaline diet is the superior choice when it comes to getting rid of and preventing illness, as well as maintaining a long and healthy life. Researchers have shown that a wide variety of illnesses may be cured entirely or prevented before they even start simply by balancing the pH level of the body with a diet that consists of the appropriate foods for optimal health. This can be done by eating foods that are alkaline and alkaline-forming.

The alkaline diets have a very straightforward method behind how they function. A higher alkaline pH level may be maintained inside the body by following a diet that consists mostly of foods that are very alkaline. Because of this, the body is able to use its own natural mechanisms to safeguard healthy cells and to maintain a healthy mineral balance, both of which are crucial to the body's ability to operate properly. Because fasting may create changes in the body's hormone levels, this is of utmost significance for those who utilise fasting as a method of weight loss or maintenance. The alkaline diet will assist in preserving the body's natural hormone balance and will help individuals maintain a healthy weight.

The body will try to adjust to a high level of acidity in a number of different ways, one of which is by putting on excessive weight. Simply being alive results in the production of acid by human beings. When individuals eat a diet that is high in beverages and foods that produce acid, the body's inherent capacity to adjust to changes in diet is overwhelmed and harmed as a result. In the event that the acids are not eliminated from the body through the waste products, the body will start to store the acids in the fatty tissue if this continues.

The elimination of waste items via the production of urine is one of the primary roles of the kidneys. One of these waste products is an excess of acid in the body. There are hormones in the body that will operate to assist the kidneys in their process of eliminating excess acid. One of these hormones is known as cortisol. One of the primary contributors of visceral fat in the body, which is caused by excess fat reserves, is the stress hormone cortisol. This is the kind of fat that gathers around the internal organs of the body and stores itself there. In addition to this, it causes extra fat to be stored in the abdominal region.

The generation of cortisol by the body is hampered by the fact that it does not always take place at the precise moment when it is required the most. When the brain detects that the body is under stress, such as when a person is being physically assaulted, the adrenal glands will release an increased quantity of the chemicals cortisol and adrenaline. This is because the brain tells the adrenal glands that the body is under stress. The issue is that the brain is unable to differentiate between true stress that is immediate in nature and stress that is generated by other issues in the body. This is the source of the problem. An assault on one's person would undoubtedly result in emotions of tension. However, there are things that people do to themselves that may cause the body to feel stressed to the point where it will generate an excessive quantity of cortisol. The following are some examples of these:

Excessive exertion

Having a weight problem

Struggling to walk due to the negative effects of heavy weight on the joints

Inability to get a good breath due to carrying too much extra weight

Unhealthy levels of blood pressure

underlying medical conditions such as diabetes and renal disease

The list may be endlessly expanded. The main idea here is that anything that causes the body to experience stress will lead the body to generate excessive levels of cortisol, more than what is required for cells to perform at their absolute best.

The body uses cortisol for a specific purpose. In order for the human body to function properly, this chemical component is required. Cortisol has a role in the regulation of energy by helping to decide whether the body should get its fuel from protein, fat, or carbohydrates. Each and every cell in the body has a cortisol receptor, which allows the cortisol molecules to provide the cells with the kind of food that contains the energy that the cells need. In addition to this, cortisol reduces the amount of insulin that is produced by the pancreas. Insulin's duty is to utilise the sugar from the food that we eat to store it in our bodies so that we may use it later for energy. Cortisol would prefer that the sugar be used up right now, and it works to prevent insulin from storing an excessive amount of sugar in the body. When there is a need for glucose in the cells as a source of energy, cortisol is the hormone that steps in to provide it.

When there is an excess of the stress hormone cortisol in the body, as there is when there is stress, problems begin to arise. Keep in mind that the body is unable to differentiate between genuine stress brought on by an external factor and the tension that is produced as a result of engaging in unhealthy behaviours. This results in the ongoing production of more cortisol by the body. After then, the pancreas produces more insulin in order to combat the effects of the cortisol. Cortisol is the only hormone that the cells of the body react to after they have stopped responding to insulin. This causes the body to store extra fat in locations where it should not store excess fat because it causes the cells to stop responding to insulin. The pancreas quits generating insulin, the amount of sugar in the bloodstream rises and remains elevated, and the individual gets type 2 diabetes in conjunction with being overweight. Both of these disorders lead the body to produce an ever-increasing quantity of acid, which the body therefore has trouble getting rid of and must work hard to do so.

A Rundown Of The Buffering Systems Found In The Body

The body's buffering mechanisms are responsible for its defence against waste products that are acidic. The consumption of acidic foods and the activity of the metabolism both contribute to the waste. A material is said to be buffered when it is brought into contact with an opposing substance in order to neutralise both of them. When alkali and acid combine, the resulting substance is neutralised, also known as buffered.

The buffering systems of the body may be found both inside and outside of individual cells, as well as in the blood and other biological fluids. The bicarbonate, phosphate, and protein buffers are the buffering systems that are found in the blood. The lungs, the kidneys, and the skin are the organs that act as buffers in the body. Urination is how the kidneys get rid of excess acid in the body, making them one of the most essential organs for this process. The degree of acidity in the body may be determined by looking at the pH level of the urine.

The amino acid glutamine serves as an additional essential buffer in the body. Within the muscular tissue, glutamine is the amino acid that is most prevalent. A high use of glutamine for buffering purposes might result in the breakdown of muscle tissue at times of increased acidity.

The process of buffering involves the use of alkaline minerals. Calcium and magnesium are the two that are considered to be the most vital. The bones are where calcium and magnesium are found; the muscles and bones together are where magnesium is found.

The significance of calcium in the body

Acidic waste can only be buffered to a certain extent by the organs (kidneys, lungs, and skin) on a regular basis. Calcium, which is the body's primary buffering mineral, is used in an effort by the body to neutralise the effects of high acid loading. On the other hand, if after all of this work there is still any acid waste left behind, it has to be turned into solid trash. The excess acid that the kidneys are unable to eliminate combines with calcium and is converted into a salt that has no taste or odour. The pH level of the body's fluids cannot be altered by this salt since it has been neutralised. It is not possible for it to make the blood or any other fluids more acidic. However, this salt will need to be kept in a secure location. Calcification is the term that describes this process. This is the first step in the development of kidney stones, gout, uric acid, cholesterol plaques, and arthritis.

Step 7: Establish an Atmosphere That Encourages Success

In this book, we have already covered two different techniques for holding ourselves accountable: maintaining a food diary and creating objectives. We are going to construct a support system right now.

Establish a Party Responsible for Accountability

Along the way to living a better life, you're going to need the assistance of individuals who can keep you accountable. Keeping yourself focused and motivated is going to be much easier if you put yourself in an atmosphere that is empowering. Taking responsibility for your actions will highlight any instances in which you go off course.

In order for your group to function, you just need one or two other individuals. It won't cost you anything, and it's been shown to make it easier for people to lead healthy lives. There is no valid reason for you not to establish a peer-to-peer accountability group.

Find a small group of individuals that have the same objectives as you do and make that your first step. You have to make an effort, if at all feasible, to locate buddies or family members who share your objectives. You want to surround yourself with individuals who won't be scared to tell you the truth if they think you're slacking off.

Make sure to schedule weekly meetings or 'check ins'. Attend these gatherings in person whenever it is at all feasible. Having said that, some of you may have schedules that make it impossible for you to get together in person every week; in that case, you might create a virtual environment for yourself, such as a Facebook Group or a Skype conversation.

Establish some kind of framework for your organisation. It's not only a chance to hang out and make new friends when you join an accountability group. I'm not suggesting that you shouldn't enjoy yourself, but you really need to work for something. Talk about what you've achieved, the challenges you've faced, and how you intend to bounce back from those obstacles.

How to Come Up with Recipes for an Alkaline Diet

This step is by far the most straightforward of the whole procedure. You have gained all of the necessary knowledge on which meals you should eat and which foods you should steer clear of from the previous chapters. Find the recipes for the meals you like most after first deciding which of these foods you favour. As you go through the alkaline diet, you should begin experimenting with different recipes until you reach the point where you can make your own.

Take into consideration the macronutrients while you work on the recipes. Keep in mind that you do not need to consume dairy products in order to get calcium, nor do you need to consume meat in order to get protein. Earlier in the book, you gained knowledge about potential alternatives that are derived from plants.

If you want to create your own recipes, the most essential thing to keep in mind is that you need to be passionate about the food that you prepare. You might, for instance, substitute almond milk with coconut milk if you don't like for the flavour of almond milk. If you do not like tomatoes, you can simply leave them out of the recipe. In this aspect, the alkaline diet offers a reasonable amount of leeway.

Get a binder, and get started compiling your very own assortment of culinary creations. When you start to construct your weekly meal plans with this information in mind, things will go much more smoothly for you. You should make particular notes on the dishes or meals that you like the most so that you may include them in your weekly routine.

Think about becoming a member of a few different alkaline diets groups either online or on social media. Talking to others who have experience with this diet will not only lead to the discovery of more incredible dishes, but it will also provide you with the opportunity to pick up pointers and strategies that will make the process of preparing your meals much less difficult. Naturally, having some help during this time of transition from your previous diet to this one will make the process go much more quickly and easily for you.

Make the transition to a vegan or vegetarian lifestyle slowly if you decide to go that route, as many people who follow the alkaline diet ultimately do. Take into consideration executing this second transfer some time between two and four months from now. This not only makes things simpler, but it also gives you the ability to modify your recipes as required.

Calories and macronutrients may be found here.

When it comes to adhering to an alkaline diet, one thing that many people are worried about is whether or not they are receiving a enough amount of calories and nutrients. This is because the alkaline diet excludes a wide variety of foods. On the other hand, as you discovered in the chapters before this one, the foods that you can consume may provide your body with more than it requires. Consuming a wide variety of meals on a daily basis is essential.

Get a physical examination before beginning the diet. This will tell you the current state of your health and whether or not you have any vitamin deficits that have existed in the past. With this knowledge, you will be able to more accurately assess the requirements of your body and increase your consumption of foods that are rich in the nutrients that will lead to an improvement in its condition.

Calculating your basal metabolic rate is the first step in determining how many calories you need to consume each day. You will not be able to exist without these calories. After that, think about your age, how active you are, how much you weigh, and what gender you are. This will result in an increase in the total amount of basic calories. You may find calculators online that will provide you with a rough estimate of the amount of calories you should strive to consume. If one of your objectives for utilising the alkaline diet is to lose weight, once you have a solid understanding of what your body requires, you will be in a position to make reductions that are both healthy and effective.

The rest of this section is going to be devoted to discussing macronutrients. When you are developing recipes, be sure to keep a close check on them so that you can determine whether or not you are receiving the appropriate quantities.

One of the most important macronutrients is protein. The majority of individuals receive this vitamin through the foods they consume, namely meat and dairy products. However, as you well know, there are a variety of plant-based meals that contain enough amounts of protein; thus, as long as you keep your diet varied, you will be able to satisfy the requirements that your body has set for you. It is recommended that you consume an average of 0.32 grammes of this vitamin for every pound that you weigh. You will need to recalculate this figure every time your weight shifts by 10 pounds.

Your digestive system, blood sugar, ability to control hunger, and ability to maintain a healthy weight all benefit greatly from adequate consumption of fibre. The fact that the foods on the alkaline diet are, for the most part, high in fibre is one of their many positive aspects. A side benefit of consuming insoluble fibre is that it helps maintain a pH equilibrium in the digestive tract. Additionally, there contains soluble fibre, which is the kind of fibre that helps regulate blood sugar and is beneficial to digestion.

We will now move on to carbohydrates. It is to your advantage to adhere to this diet precisely because it will allow you to consume a greater proportion of complex carbs. Because you are restricting your diet to whole foods, the amount of simple carbs you consume should be maintained to a minimum. Maintaining a healthy level of energy throughout the day is much easier when you consume an adequate amount of complex carbohydrates. since of this, you won't have to worry about not receiving enough of an essential nutrient like fibre since these foods often include significant levels of it.

The alkaline diet places a significant emphasis on eating healthy fats. You'll discover that foods like avocado are commonplace, and that these meals are rich with the fats that your body needs to function properly. When you consume the appropriate types of fats and refrain from consuming trans fats, this leads to a better cardiovascular system, which in turn contributes to an improvement in overall well-being. Saturated fat is a kind of fat that should be consumed in moderation but may be consumed in small amounts. One example of this would be the presence of it in coconut oil. Your main priority should be monounsaturated fats. Avocado, some nuts, and healthy oils are all good sources of this nutrient. It is advised that you consume a diet high in polyunsaturated fats as long as the food in question has not been processed.

Even though it's not a macronutrient, staying hydrated is incredibly essential as well. When you are well hydrated, you will have less cravings. In addition to this, it makes sure that your body gets all of the water it needs to carry out its functions. The majority of alkaline recipes call for items that have a high proportion of water, and it is recommended that about 80 percent of the water you consume come from your diet. The following are a few recipes for infused water that will make it simpler to keep hydrated.

What Is Meant By The Term "Alkalized Water," And How Exactly May Drinking It Improve Our Health?

To start, it's important to comprehend the fact that water is a need for all forms of life.

Water makes up three quarters of our bodies and serves as the medium for a wide variety of reactions that are essential to maintaining life in the human body. Due to water's exceptional capacity as a solvent, it is often either the reactant or the product in a number of important chemical processes that take place within the body.

Ionised water is another name for alkalized water, which is another frequent name. The chemical formula for water is expressed as "H_2O," where the hydrogen atoms are considered positive and the OH molecules are considered negative. Because it contains an equal amount of hydrogen and hydroxide ions, natural, unadulterated water is considered to be neutral or inert.

Alkaline water has a higher concentration of hydroxide ions in their normal state, which are used by our cells. When compared to regular water, alkaline water contains around one hundred times the amount of oxygen and has a pH value that ranges from 8 to 10. Most significantly, this alkalinity is accomplished without the use of any hazardous chemicals in any part of the production process.

Not only is there an elevation in pH, but the molecules of water are also reassembled into a form that is less complicated, has more positive effects, and is easier for the body to ingest.

The Advantages of Drinking Alkaline Water

Detoxification of harmful substances

In layman's terms, free radicals are atoms or molecules that, by their very nature, exhibit high levels of reactivity. They come into being as a result of the reaction of oxygen with certain molecules.

Because it contains so many antioxidants, drinking alkalized water may assist the body in developing a greater capacity to rid itself of harmful free radicals. The increased production of antioxidants also contributes to a quicker healing process for wounds and scars.

Increased levels of Hydration
Ionisation is a process that helps break up large clusters of water into smaller ones, making the water simpler for the blood to absorb. The circulation of blood is improved by alkalized water, which also has the ability to permeate locations with high levels of acidity. Your skin begins to glow and feel more soft after using this product.

Put a stop to the process of becoming older.
It is well established that an accumulation of acidic by-products has a speeding effect on the ageing process. The accumulation of waste products

leads to organ damage, which accelerates the natural ageing process of the body's interior.

lactic acid, carbonic acid, fatty acids, and ammonia are all examples of waste products that are acidic. The acidic properties of trash may be neutralised by alkaline minerals.

Containment of Allergic Reactions

Stress, an unhealthy diet, and an inability to maintain a regular exercise routine may all cause changes in the pH level of the body. Reduced tolerance to allergic reactions is one of the consequences of a pH that is out of whack. Consuming water that has been alkalized on a regular basis may help protect against allergic reactions.

Enhanced Condition of the Hair and Skin

Acne and other skin irritations respond well to treatment with alkalized water. It is able to remove grease, oil, and dirt without the use of harsh chemicals, and it does it very effectively. In addition to that, it assists in calming skin that is dry, itchy, and chapped.

Enhanced Flavour and Gastronomic Experience
In order to neutralise the acidic effects of things like cooking and brewing coffee with alkalized water, etc.

Excellent for use in gardening
The use of water that has been alkalized is a great way to neutralise soils that are too acidic. Additionally, alkalized water is effective for the germination of seedlings and may be used in the production of insecticides.
Other advantages associated with consuming alkalized water include stronger immune systems (greater resistance to cancer) and enhanced absorption of minerals, which leads to improved health, energy, and stamina levels. Alkalized water may also be used to reduce acidity levels in the body.

Smoothie Made With Orange Creamsicle

INGREDIENTS:

- 1 teaspoonofsweetener
- 1 tablespoonofvanillaextract
- 2 cookie-typemaria
- 1 teaspoonorangezest
- 1 naturalskimmedyogurtorvanillaflavor (canbereplacedbyvanillaicecreamball s)
- 150 ml oforangejuice

INSTRUCTIONS

With the assistance of a blender, you may make a cookie batter using orange juice.

The next step is to include the vanilla extract, orange zest, strained yoghurt, and sweetener into the mixture. You could use vanilla ice cream in place of the yoghurt, and the end product would still be rather decadent.

Combine all of the ingredients in a mixing bowl and beat them together until the mixture is smooth and creamy.

If you want to have a really cold experience with it, add some ice cubes to it.

Serve in glasses and garnish with fresh mint leaves or a pinch each of cocoa and orange zest. You may also sprinkle with a teaspoon of cocoa or orange zest.

The best course of action is to consume it right away so that it does not lose its freshness or suffer any degradation in its qualities. In any other case, store in the refrigerator until it is time to eat.

This orange cream hake is not only appetising, but it is also quite nutritious when considered from any angle. Do not put off preparing it at home any longer! You will be able to provide your family with a natural and nutritious option while just using a small number of ingredients and without incurring significant additional costs.

Green And Herbal Loose Leaf Teas Should Be Consumed Regularly.

Consuming whole leaf teas is one of the most effective methods to naturally cleanse the body and maintain good health. There are numerous different natural remedies that may help you maintain your health. If you are not going to juice and drink the tincture every day (which I strongly urge you do), then drinking tea is the next and most critical step in the process.

You need to be willing to do things that the majority of people won't in order to maintain your health. Since the typical person consumes coffee (which, in moderation and without added sugar, might be beneficial to your health), you can only image what the minority of healthy individuals are doing to stay that way.

Teas are among some of the healthiest things on the world, and they supply tough trace nutrients that you truly are not receiving from an industrialised diet. If you drink tea, you should drink it often. Even teas that have been processed are healthier for you than beverages like soda or energy drinks.

The majority of teas (whole leaf, unprocessed) include: Teas contain potent polyphenols, which are rated as one of the most potent antioxidants that can be found anywhere. Teas are unprocessed.

If you drink only three to five glasses of water every day, you may reduce your risk of having a heart attack, stroke, and other connected disorders.

The body is better able to metabolise fats thanks to the effects of tea, and it also stores less fat.

➤There is a correlation between tea consumption and extreme longevity, and civilizations that consume a lot of tea tend to have people who live the longest.

Get started right now on drinking herbal teas made from long leaf.

The fourth step is to eat your way to a higher alkalinity.

The sensation that you are missing out on something important is one of the most challenging aspects of dieting. This will alter if you offer superfoods as healthy snacks instead of junk food.

Consuming healthy snacks that are also alkaline may do wonders for reducing the size of your waistline. Studies have also shown a connection between snacking on healthful foods, such as nuts with the skins still on them, and living a longer life.

Put sugar out of your mind! Start munching on high-quality, organic whole foods like: Nuts of all types — these foods tend to have a pH that is neutral, but nonetheless, they are very excellent for you. Fruits and vegetables that are grown without pesticides. Snacks that contribute to an increase in health include a hand full of almonds, a cup of berries, or a serving of dense greens.

You may make some of the greatest snacks by preparing them in advance and having them ready to go at a moment's notice, and some of the best snacks include vividly coloured vegetables and fresh citrus. Again, foods that are completely organic, such as citrus, may seem to be overly acidic to consume, but the components from which they are generated work in conjunction with your body to naturally bring the pH level down.

Despite the fact that there is a great deal of controversy around alkaline water, an increasing number of medical professionals are coming around to its benefits. It is possible to immediately lower your pH by drinking alkaline water with a pH of 9-11; but, in order to retain it at that level, you will also need to consume alkaline meals. Drinking distilled water is safest, but you should still check with a medical professional if you have any concerns.

You are eliminating the bulk of unhealthy food options from your new lifestyle, so if you maintain nibbling on these things and water, you will make tremendous progress since you are reducing the overall number of unhealthy food options.

The Link Between an Acidic Diet and Osteoporosis

Osteoporosis is a degenerative bone disease that is characterised by a reduction in bone mineral content. This decrease in bone mineral content leads to decreased bone density and strength as well as an increased risk of breaking a bone.

In order to neutralise the acids that are produced by eating an acidic diet, proponents of the alkaline diet believe that the body draws alkaline minerals like calcium from the bones. This is done in order to keep the blood pH at a consistent level. As was already said, this is not even close to being accurate. It is not the bones but rather the kidneys and the respiratory system that are in charge of maintaining the pH of the blood.

In point of fact, a great number of studies have shown that increasing the consumption of animal protein is beneficial for bone metabolism. This is because it leads to an increase in calcium retention and it activates IGF-1, which is an insulin-like growth factor that promotes bone regeneration. As a result, the concept that bone loss might be caused by an acidic diet is not supported by scientific evidence.

Acidic Diet and the Breakdown of Muscle

In order to get rid of the extra acid brought on by an acidic diet, proponents of the alkaline diet think that the kidneys would take amino acids from muscle tissues in order to get rid of the excess acid. Amino acids are the fundamental building blocks of protein. The postulated process is somewhat comparable to that which is responsible for osteoporosis.

As was previously said, the kidneys and lungs, and not the muscles, are responsible for regulating the pH of the blood. Therefore, the use of acidic foods such as meat, dairy products, and eggs does not lead to a reduction in muscle mass. In point of fact, they are complete proteins found in foods, which means that they will assist repair damaged muscle tissue and stop the loss of muscle mass.

What Kinds of Food Did Our Ancestors Consume?

Whether or if our pre-agricultural ancestors had net acidic or net alkaline diets has been the subject of investigation in a number of studies. They made the very surprising discovery that around half of the hunter-gatherers consumed meals that were net acid-forming, whereas the other half consumed diets that were net alkaline-forming.

The more inhospitable the climate, the more animal proteins individuals consumed in their diets. Diets high in acid-forming foods became increasingly prevalent as people travelled farther north of the equator. Their diet grew more alkaline as they moved into more tropical regions where there was an abundance of fruits and vegetables.

The hypothesis that cancer, osteoporosis, and atrophy of muscular tissue are caused by eating acidic foods or diets high in protein is not sound from the point of view of evolutionary biology. Although one half of the hunter-gatherers had diets that were net acid-forming, there was no indication that either group suffered from degenerative illnesses.

It is important to note that there is no diet that is universally effective for all people. This is one of the reasons why metabolic typing is so beneficial in selecting the diet that is most appropriate for you. Because we all have somewhat different genetic make-ups, some individuals will reap the benefits of an acidic diet, some will get the benefits of an alkaline diet, and others will reap the benefits of both. This is the origin of the proverb that states "one man's food can be another man's poison."

It is a fact that the majority of individuals who make the move to an alkaline diet report considerable benefits in their health. Be that as it may, keep in mind that there might be other factors at play here: * The vast majority of us do not consume nearly enough fruits and vegetables. The Centre for Disease Control and Prevention reports that just 9% of Americans consume an adequate amount of veggies and only 13% consume an adequate amount of fruits. If you transition to an alkaline diet, you will naturally consume more veggies and fruits than if you were eating a more acidic diet. After all, they include a significant quantity of phytochemicals, antioxidants, and fibre, all of which are important components of a healthy diet. When you increase the amount of veggies and fruits you eat, you probably also reduce the amount of processed meals you consume.

* Those who are lactose intolerant or who have a food sensitivity to eggs, both of which are very prevalent among the general population, will benefit by reducing the amount of dairy and eggs they consume in their diet. Those who are gluten-sensitive, have leaky gut syndrome, or an autoimmune condition will benefit from reducing the amount of grains in their diet.

Rejuvenating tonic, relaxing, reduces anxiousness, and improves immune system health are some of the uses for this herb.

The arrangement, in addition to the prescriptions:

To make a cup of tea, bring one teaspoon of dried and sliced root to a simmer in one cup of water or milk for ten minutes. The tension. Consume something to drink once or twice every day.

Normalised Extract (25 percent with the anode): Consume 500 milligrammes two or three times on a daily basis.

The Black Cohosh herb

Utilisations: Eases menstrual cramping and joint pain, and is often used to alleviate the symptoms of menopause as well.

The arrangement, as well as the dosages:

Tincture: consume 12 millilitres three times each day.

Take 2080 mg twice day, as directed by the normalised extract.

Calendula flower

Utilisations: Calendula has been used for some time to quiet irritation in the mouth, throat, and stomach. It is also widely recognised as a topical cream or balm to relieve rashes and disturbances, as well as to assist in the healing of wounds.

 Preparedness and appropriate dosages:

To make tea, pour one cup of boiling water over two teaspoons of petals. Wait ten minutes before drinking. The tension. Make a cup of tea with variations, or use it as a mouthwash or rinse.

Use the balm on your skin anywhere between two and three times each day.

Nip of catnip.

Uses include calming an upset stomach and reducing feelings of anxiety and tension in the body.

The composition and distribution of:

To make tea, pour one cup of boiling water over four to five fresh leaves or one teaspoon of dried leaves. Steep for a total of five minutes. When necessary, subject to further strain and improvement. Consume something to drink once or twice every day.

Raspberry sylvestre

Utilisations: The most effective herb for reducing the symptoms of premenstrual syndrome.

The arrangement, as well as the doses:

Capsules: Take one capsule containing 250–500 milligrammes of a dried organic product once day.

Tincture: take 23 millilitres first thing in the morning.

Cranberry is a.

Utilisations: Well-established therapy for lowering the risk of bladder illness; may also be beneficial for recurrent cases of prostatitis.

The arrangement, in addition to the prescriptions:

Juice: You should have half a cup twice a day.

Capsules: Take 300–500 mg of the concentrated juice on its own, twice day.

Stewed Zucchini With A Sour Flavour

Ingredients:

½ cup freshly squeezed tomato juice

2 tsp of Italian seasoning, organic

½ tsp of salt

2 tbsp of olive oil

4 medium-sized zucchini, peeled and sliced

1 large eggplant, peeled and chopped

3 medium-sized red bell peppers

Preparation:

Olive oil, to the tune of two teaspoons, should be spread around the bottom of a big pan. Next, include sliced zucchini and eggplant, red peppers and tomato juice into the dish. After giving it a thorough stir, season it with salt and Italian seasoning. One last whisk, and then add in about a half cup of water.

Prepare the dish for 15 minutes with the heat set at medium. The courgette should be easily pierced with a fork but should not be overdone.

Take the food out of the saucepan and put it in the fridge to cool. To be served chilled.

Porridge Made With Alkaline Oats And Toppings

Ingredients

1 tablespoon sunflower seeds

½ tsp cinnamon

½ tsp turmeric

250 ml almond milk

4 tbsp. organic oat flakes

½ tbsp poppy seeds

1 tablespoon linseed

Fresh or dried fruit to taste

Add coconut flakes, almonds or other nuts if desired.

Preparation:

To begin, pour the almond milk into a saucepan. Then, stir in the ground cinnamon and turmeric, along with the oat flakes, poppy seeds, flax seeds, and sunflower seeds.

Now bring all of the ingredients to a simmer in the saucepan, but make sure they don't boil! After that, let it to cool down and swell for around ten minutes.

The completed porridge should then be transferred to a bowl. Include some fruits or nuts of your choosing as a garnish for the breakfast.

Muesli Made With Soaked Almonds And Seeds

Ingredients

1 cup unsweetened almond milk
¼ cup raw pumpkin seeds
¼ cup raw almonds
Sweetener, to taste

Cinnamon, to taste
1 tablespoon flaxseeds
1 tablespoon chia seeds

Directions

In a bowl, combine all of the ingredients, then season with cinnamon and a sweetener of your choice.

Soak it up over the night, then have more in the morning.

Green Drink That Is Alkalizing.

Ingredients:

- 2 inches piece ginger, peeled, sliced
- 2 tablespoons chia seeds, soaked in water overnight if possible
- 2 teaspoons flaxseed oil
- Juice of 2 lemons
- Stevia drops to taste
- 2 avocados, peeled, pitted, chopped
- 2 cups coconut water
- 1 small continental cucumber, chopped
- 1/2 cup fresh mint leaves
- 1 cup fresh parsley
- 4 medium kale leaves, discard hard stems and ribs, torn

Method:

Put all of the ingredients into a blender and process until the mixture is completely smooth.

Place the liquid in large glasses.

Prepare with crushed ice and serve.

Corn Syrup With A High Fructose Content

You have almost certainly seen the substance high fructose corn syrup before, or at the very least, you have seen it listed as an ingredient on the packaging of some of your go-to snacks or fast meals. In spite of the fact that this was created using actual maize in the processing stage, the final product bears no resemblance to maize whatsoever. When all is said and done, high fructose corn syrup and refined sugar are functionally equivalent to one another. Its primary function is as a sweetener, and it may be found in meals such as soda, cereal, and several other sweet and convenient items. This component is used often as a result of the fact that the price per unit is substantially lower than that of sugar, and it is also much simpler to deal with.

Colouring Agents in Food

In processed foods, a wide variety of various food colorings are employed to give them the aesthetic appeal that will make them seem appetising and make people purchase them. This will encourage consumers to buy the processed meals. The issue here is that these colours are made up of chemicals that we do not have any business putting into our bodies and that are known to be the root cause of hyperactivity in children. After all of the processing and adding of chemicals, and before they have been coloured, these dyes are added in mass-produced meals since, without them, the majority of these processed foods would seem extremely unpleasant and of a grayish-brown colour. For instance, the majority of the time, when we see the words "brown bread" printed on a packaging, we automatically assume that this indicates that the product is better for our health. This is not always the case, however, since brown bread may sometimes be nothing more than white bread or bread made with processed wheat and a number of chemicals that has been dyed brown to make it seem to customers like us that it is better for our health.

Chemicals used as preservatives

Because there are so many distinct names for preservatives and because there are so many various types of preservatives, only the most highly trained scientists are able to properly pronounce them. Preservatives are substances that are put into food in order to extend its freshness or to make it last longer on the market. Consider the possibility that you have come across movies or articles on highly processed foods that make light of the fact that after twenty years they will still seem exactly the same and will not have developed any mould or deteriorated in any way. In such a scenario, the reason for this is because preservatives were added to it. When something has a longer shelf life, extra preservatives are often added to it to ensure its integrity. If you often purchase fruit or vegetables, you probably already know that after about a week or two in the refrigerator, they will begin to develop mould and rot. This is a natural process. This is something that a whole, natural food would do, but something that a product that has been industrially processed would not accomplish.

Salt, sweetener, and fatty foods

Now for the trifecta: fat, salt, and sugar are sometimes considered to be a triad in the foods that have been the most processed. Even if you believe a dish, like a french fry from a fast food restaurant, to be excessively salty, there is almost certainly a significant amount of sugar added to it. Although the combination of these three makes for a pleasing flavour for our taste senses, it is not very beneficial to the body in any way. When they are all combined in a single food item, it causes your body to have a recurring need for those components as well as that meal. As was said before, it is possible to find a combination of fat, salt, and sugar in products such as High-Fructose Corn

Syrup or in oils that have been hydrogenated or severely processed. Because of their low cost and high potential for flavour, these two components are used in almost all of the products that are sold in quick-service restaurants or that have undergone extensive processing. If you go to a typical restaurant where you sit down for your meal, they could not solely use items that have been prepared in factories. In spite of this, they will make it a point to combine a significant quantity of sugar, fat, and salt in a single dish. This is because they know that this is the secret to making the food taste amazing and keeping customers coming back for more.

Why Do These Foods Have Such a Strong Hold on Us?

After going through the substances that are most often used in the production of industrial meals, we will now examine the addictive qualities of these compounds, as well as the chemicals and physiological processes inside the body that are responsible for producing this effect.

To start, we are going to circle back around to casein, which is an element produced from milk that has extremely addictive qualities. In terms of its capacity to produce addiction, casein has been likened to nicotine. It is often found in cheese, which is why there is growing evidence that individuals may get addicted to cheese, and many already are. It is also the case that many people already are hooked to cheese. This occurs naturally throughout the digestive process. When cheese and other meals that include casein are digested, the casein in those foods is broken down, and one of the compounds that it breaks down into is a chemical that is very similar to opioids. This compound may be found in cheese and other foods that contain casein. Painkillers include this chemical, which has a significant potential for addiction.

It has been shown that combining fat and carbs in meals, including potato chips, pizza, french fries, and other similar items, makes these foods even more difficult to resist than other foods that do not include these same combinations of fat and carbohydrates.

It has also been shown that high-fructose corn syrup has a strong addictive potential. In terms of its addictive potential, this chemical is somewhat comparable to cocaine.

The chemical composition of these meals is the root cause of their addictive properties. A chemical structure may be thought of as the arrangement of the molecules that contribute to the overall makeup of anything. Everything has a unique chemical structure, which may be thought of as a unique arrangement of molecules; this is what differentiates one item from another, while some objects have similarities in their chemical structures. If the chemical structures of two different things are very similar to one another, then the substances, materials, or objects that the two things are will be highly similar to one another. Therefore, these highly addictive compounds that may be found in industrially manufactured foods have a molecular structure that is quite comparable to the chemical structure of highly addictive substances such as cocaine, heroin, or opioids. Either this, or they break down in our digestive system, and then this process generates compounds that are extremely similar to the chemical structure of narcotics that are very addictive. Either way, the process is highly addicting. Therefore, in order to comprehend the rationale behind why these particular chemical compounds are addictive, we will have to get a deeper comprehension of the scientific workings of our brains. In the next section, we will go into this topic more to better understand why humans are so prone to developing food addictions, particularly to certain specific categories of foods.

On The Alkaline Diet, What Kinds Of Foods May I Consume?

In this section, we will discuss the foods that are acceptable for consumption on the Alkaline Diet. As we have endeavoured to impress upon you all through this electronic book, eating solid fundamentally soluble food sources is the way to progress on the Alkaline Diet. This implies eating fundamental debris food varieties (80% of your eating regimen) and generally staying away from corrosive debris food sources (the remaining 20% of your dietary total).

Consider the caustic debris dietary sources to be your own kryptonite. Acid waste food varieties can upset your body to the point of causing or fueling fundamental medical conditions, cause you to feel less active, and possibly even put you in danger for serious medical conditions in the future and cause faster ageing. This is analogous to how kryptonite was capable of incapacitating

Superman to the point where he was unable to defeat his adversaries. I'll keep my mouth shut for your own good, but you don't need that. You must assume the identity of Superman, you must assume the identity of Captain America, and you must assume the identity of Aquaman. You need to have a lot of vitality and strength, and you need to be in good health to the point where you can tackle any task that you need to go on.

It's possible that many of you are already familiar with the concept of so-called superfoods. For those of you who are not familiar, superfoods are healthy, ordinary food kinds that include cell reinforcements and other synthetic chemicals that may help you fight illness and prevent illness. These foods have been given the name "superfoods." According to certain studies, they may have a higher life expectancy. You may find out what some of these superfoods are by doing a search on the internet. Some examples of these foods are mango, coconut, kale, chia, avocado, salmon, garlic, and the list continues on.

Although many of you won't be familiar with the basic debris food kinds just yet, those of you who are will notice that the list of these usual superfoods includes several soluble debris food varieties, including coconut, avocado, and garlic.

Although there are some on there that we would consider corrosive trash, like fish, there are also those that are not.

The main point to take away from this is that, despite the fact that we might consider antacid debris food sources to be "superfoods" due to the fact that the vast majority of them have been shown to present a few useful benefits that can assist us with living longer, these foods are not actually comparable to the superfoods that you might have read about on the internet.

You need to use extreme caution in this situation. You must consume food sources that are classified as soluble debris rather than merely eating food kinds that are portrayed as "superfoods." Now that we've come this far, we should go right into the list of foods that neutralise acidity in the body.

To be alkaline Chart of Ashes Food

THE FRUITS

Mandarin oranges Bananas

Sweet cherries

Pina coladas Fruits: Peaches and Avocados The date(s)

Figs

Grapes Melon Fruits

Papea y papaya

New Zealand Gooseberries

Pommes d'Or

To pears

A type of sultana

Mangos are used here.

Citrus Reticulata Citrus: lemons

Lime slices

Melon, Watermelon The pomegranate fruit Cucurbitapepo

Tomatoes and radishes both.

It's a cauliflower.

Kale

Kelp

Collard Greens with Wakame

Onions with Chives

Endive Chard Endive

Sprouts of the Brussels

OILS FRUITS AND VEGETABLES NUTS AND SEEDS Carrots /

Corn

Various types of Mushrooms

Carrots Cabbage

Peas

Potatoes baked in their skins (skin alone)

The olives

Cauliflower Sweet Potato Zucchini

Bibb lettuce

The celery and the beets

Compress Okra and Garlic Together

Broccoli and spinach, please.

Garlic Onions Parsley

The asparagus

GRAINS AND BEANS (AND MORE)

The grain quinoa

Millet Rice with Wild Rice

The amaranth plant.

The soy bean

Beans, or Green Gluten and yeast both

The GRASSES

Oil extracted from Avocado Coconut Oil Olive Oil Flax Seed Oil Olive Oil Flax Seed Oil

Oil from Canola Toasted almonds

The chestnuts

Cocos de mer

Seeds of the Sunflower The seeds of sesame Seeds of the Pumpkin Seeds of flax

Grass Shaves Made From Oat Dog de Grass barley grass, kamut grass, and other types of grass Grass of wheat

DAIRY products

Silken Tofu

Milk from a Goat Lactose-Free Breast Milk Whey

SUGARY PRODUCTS Honey and sugar in their raw form

Toasted Maple Syrup

The Syrup of Rice

Stevia and other forms of tofu

Tea with Ginger

Teas Including Green Tea and Herbal Teas

Mint

Menthapiperita

Pasta made from buckwheat To be alkaline The water Kraut or sauerkraut

These were your primary sources of food from trash, and while it may be evident that there are a huge lot of them, you shouldn't worry too much since following this diet isn't like being thrown into a prison in a foreign nation. You may without a doubt develop a meal plan for the day that will successfully enable you to prepare each of your dinners at home using components acquired from your nearby grocery store or rancher's market. This is something that is completely doable. In the event that this is really important to you, you may actually eat out. You will have a lot of options to choose from! The corrosive debris food sources are the next on the list (of the competing group), which we will now examine. While following the Alkaline Diet, you should limit your consumption of these specific types of foods. 6. A Bowl of Healthy Green Smoothies

Including avocado in your diet is a great way to get more antioxidants, such glutathione, as well as fibre, which both assist your body in detoxing and flushing out toxins. In addition to being high in monounsaturated fats, avocado is also a good source of alkaline minerals such as magnesium and potassium.

Assists in 2 Components or Elements

1 teaspoon of toasted almond flakes

1 level tablespoon of coconut, unsweetened

Chia seeds, one teaspoon's worth

1 lime, zested and juiced

1 compact bunch of freshly chopped parsley

1 cup of spinach leaves that are fresh.

1 small cubed cucumber, peeled and seeded

1 ounce (or cup) of coconut water

1 fully ripe avocado, peeled and chopped into small pieces

the way forward

1. In a blender, combine all of the ingredients and process until they have a smooth consistency.

2. Next, pour the beverage into a bowl, and if you like, you may garnish it with chia seeds, coconut, and almonds.

3. Serve as soon as possible.

Starter's Guide To The Alkaline Diet

The study of the human body is one of the most intricate and extensive subfields that fall under the umbrella of the scientific discipline. As is common knowledge, the most complex buildings are also the ones that are the most challenging to maintain.

We have heard of numerous fitness programmes that focus on reducing the amount of sugar in the body, losing weight, and eating foods that contain the most minerals and proteins; nevertheless, the things that need to be taken care of go much farther than that.

The number of things that may be harmful to the body can be divided into two categories: those that have the potential to cause death to us and those that are only slightly less severe. The list of things that are important for the body and the list of things that can be harmful to it can both be divided into these two categories. The dietary concerns that are of less significance are often accorded less attention, and they are almost entirely ignored, as a result of the focus placed on the matters that are of greater significance. One of these issues is the amount of alkaline that is present in your body.

As it turns out, the degree of acidity may be determined using a scale called the PH scale, which has 14 different degrees. The scale goes from level 1 to level 7 in a decreasing sequence of acidity, with level 1 being the most acidic of the seven levels.

The scale becomes neutral at level 7, and from level 7 to level 14, it runs in rising order of alkalinity, with level 14 being the highest alkaline point on the scale. Because too much of anything is bad for you, nature strives to maintain a healthy balance between seemingly opposing forces, such as heat and cold, day and night, and activity and rest. This is because extremes of any kind may have negative effects.

Therefore, a measurement of the average makes the situation optimal in most cases. On the other hand, it is best for human beings to have a slightly alkaline bodily state at all times.

Given that hydrochloric acid is the fluid that can be found inside of a human stomach, one may deduce that a human stomach has a predisposition towards an acidic nature.

The body has a natural tendency to create an excessive amount of acid, which may be very harmful to the body if it is not sometimes and properly diluted with water. But is there sufficient water? Even if it has a pH level of 7, it can only partially counteract the effects of the acid that is already present in your body; hence, there is still a need for something that is more effective in combating the highly concentrated fluids. Since alkali is the opposite of acid, it serves as the ideal remedy for neutralising acidic conditions, which are dangerous and should be avoided at all costs.

The presence of an excessive amount of acid inside the body is hazardous to one's health and should not be taken lightly.

Few individuals are aware of how much of an impact this has on them in their day-to-day lives, but it has been shown through research and observation that this condition is responsible for a variety of health problems, including increased weariness and exhaustion, muscular discomfort and cramping, difficulty breathing, and running out of breath.

On a larger scale, this imbalance may be responsible for the weakening of bones, disorders of the bones, weight gain, and may provide a more favourable environment for the formation of deadly diseases such as cancer and other cardiac problems.

Despite the fact that the imbalance is alarming, there is a remedy for everything. In this particular scenario, the antidote is obviously the consumption of materials that are high in alkali. It's possible that some of you are visualising eating your laundry detergent, but thankfully, the treatment is considerably more appetising.

It is in point of fact a comprehensive eating plan that is made up mostly of fresh fruits and vegetables, as well as various kinds of dried fruits and nuts. The grains, citrus fruits, dairy products, and shellfish all contribute to the acidity of our meals, but grains are the primary source. It is also possible for it to be found in foods that have undergone extensive processing. Should we therefore refuse to consume anything that even somewhat resembles food because it could contain acid? The correct response is unquestionably not.

As was said in a previous part of this essay, the natural world is one of harmony; hence, the circumstances under which we are able to exist in this life and make the most of everything need to likewise be in appropriate proportion to one another.

The term "Alkaline diet" refers to a way of eating that includes foods that provide us with a mix of foods that are rich in alkali and foods that are proportionately acidic. This is done in order to combat the increasing acidic condition of the body.

According to research, when this diet is effective in making the body slightly more alkaline than acidic, it is able to combat common ailments such as the flu, coughing, increased mucus production, and a drop in energy levels.

It has also been shown to be effective in treating headaches and anxiety, in addition to boosting weight reduction in a healthy manner.

The alkaline diet is a win-win situation for everyone involved, but the issue that needs to be answered is: what exactly is this amazing diet? One thing that can be mentioned with absolute certainty about this diet is that the individual who is following it would be required to depend primarily on fruits and nuts and refrain from consuming very acidic foods. This is one of the things that can be said.

Carrots, cucumbers, soy beans, and lettuce are some examples of the kinds of foods that are often required to be consumed as part of a diet. Pears, bananas, and watermelons are also OK to consume, but only in moderation.

And despite the fact that it makes the most of the diet that we eat on a daily basis, we would have to avoid or, at the at least, keep under control the amount of meat, poultry, pig, fish, and dairy products that we consume whenever it is feasible. Caffeine, chocolate, and alcoholic drinks should be rigorously banned from consumption, although brown rice and fish caught in fresh water could be spared from this rule.

This alkaline diet offers us with a fantastic weapon to battle the excess acid that is already present in our body; nevertheless, this diet should not be tried on youngsters, patients with cardiac conditions, nursing or pregnant women, or those who have renal difficulties.

The general public, regardless of whether or not they are in good health, should also follow the traditional practise of seeing their nutritionist before beginning a new diet plan or intending to participate in strenuous exercise, muscle building/burning, the use of steroids, or other rigorous sports. This is important for a number of reasons.

Because the symptoms of this disorder are quite prevalent, they should not be relied upon as a means of determining the amount of acid present in the body of a patient.

Medication and diet have nothing to do with taking educated guesses, and those who are considering adopting this diet should first determine the amount of acid that is truly present in their bodies before beginning the diet.

It is safe for you to continue with this diet after it has been confirmed that you need it; nevertheless, following this diet when it is found that you do not require it may result in unfavourable situations. As the old adage goes, prevention is always preferable than treatment. And as we often emphasise, the responsibility for your health is not ours but yours.

Oat That Is Alkaline

Ingredients

- Water
- Nut Milk
- Coconut/non-dairyyoghurt
- Cinnamon (1 tspperperson)
- Handful ofmixed nuts/seeds
- Optional: berries of yourchoice
- Oats (preferably organic)
- Chia seeds (1 dessertspoon per person)
- Coconutoil (1 dessert spoon perperson)

Instructions

Essentially, you should boil your typical amount of oats in water. It wasn't milk. WATER.

Then place the chia seeds in a separate bowl and stir in the oats and water that have been brought to a simmer in the pan. Cook the mixture until it is just a little on the dry side for your taste, and then whisk in a splash or two of the nut milk (coconut milk is my favourite, but you can use any other kind of non-dairy milk).

After removing the pan from the heat, add the coconut oil, cinnamon, and a little amount of the non-dairy yoghurt, and mix to combine. After adding the nuts and seeds to the bowl, finish it off with blueberries or strawberries if you count them as part of your daily fruit intake (to reduce the amount of fructose you consume on a daily basis, I recommend eating no more than 1-2 servings of in-season fruit).

Justswappingthe 250ml of milk per person, takingout the sugar/honey, and adding in chia (omega 3 and extra fibre to supportdigestion, brain function, metabolism, heart health), coconut oil (MCT oilsformetabolism, loweringbadcholesterolandbrainfunctio n) and cinnamon (speeded metabolism, lowerbloodsugar levels, reduce heartdiseaseriskfactors) – you're turning a 'regular' breakfast into a SUPER ALKALINE BREAKFAST.

It is awesome and has been a lifesaver for me on many hectic mornings while getting myself and my family ready for work, school, or kindergarten!

Crepes Made With Buckwheat

- 1 cup buckwheat flour
- 1 tbsp. olive oil
- 3 tbsps. olive oil
- Fresh tomatoes
- 2 eggs
- ½ liter water
- ½ tsp. Celtic sea salt

Put all of the ingredients into your mixer and let the mixture a minute to be processed. In the event that you do not own a mixer, all you need to do is place the flour in a bowl and combine the eggs, oil, and Celtic salt in the same bowl. Toss everything together. Slowly pour in some water. Stir for about three minutes, or until a smooth consistency has been achieved. The combination should sit undisturbed for two hours while covered with a towel.

The next thing you need to do is put some oil into a pot. When the crepes are ready, you may begin turning them over to expose the other side. Assist in.

The Positive Effects Of An Alkaline Diet On Health

Consume Alkaline Foods to Improve Your Health.

The food that we consume now is very different from the food that our ancestors consumed, and it is also quite different from the food that we have been used to eating in modern times. That old saying is very true: "We are what we eat." The kinds of foods that we eat have caused us to fall behind the rapid pace of technological development. When you visit a grocery store, you will be astounded by the number of processed food items and animal products that are stocked in the aisles and on the shelves. There is no difficulty in locating a fast food restaurant in our neighbourhood because to the ease with which one may get fast food these days.

The introduction of whole new eating habits, such as high-protein diets, may be partially attributed to the rise in popularity of fad diets. In recent years, there has been a rise in the consumption of animal products and processed food items. This is due to the fact that an increasing number of individuals are eliminating the daily supply of fruit and vegetables from their diets.

It should not come as a surprise that these days a large number of individuals are suffering from a wide variety of illnesses and allergies, including bone diseases, heart problems, and a great deal of other conditions. Some medical professionals attribute these diseases to the meals that we choose to put in our bodies. Certain kinds of food may throw off the equilibrium in our bodies to such an extent that they can cause health issues when consumed in large enough quantities. If only we could change our eating habits, we may be able to reduce the risk of developing diseases and improve our overall health. However, this is very unlikely.

Why Maintaining an Alkaline Body PH Is Crucial Our bodies

The alkaline-to-acid ratio, which is assessed by the pH level in the body, must be in a state of equilibrium for the body to be considered healthy. pH values may vary from 0 to 14, with 7 being the point at which they are considered neutral. Any value that is lower than 7 is thought to be acidic. Refined foods, such as meat and meat derivatives, candy, and certain sweetened beverages, often cause the body to produce a significant quantity of acid. This is because the body must break down these foods.

Acidosis, which is caused by a high level of acdc in both the bloodstream and the cells of the body, is the common index for the many diseases that are now affecting a great number of individuals. Some medical experts are of the opinion that cigarette smoking is to blame for the critical illnesses that a large number of people are experiencing in today's society.

The alkaline or alkaline diet, both of which are typically present in our bodies, neutralise the high level of acidic that is present in the body in order to achieve an equilibrated state. The primary role of alkaline in the body is to do this function. However, the existence of the alkane in the body is quickly depleted due to the high amount of acid content that it needs to neutralise, and there is not enough alkaline food consumed to restore the low levels of alkane.

A Healthy Alkaline-Acid Balance Is Necessary for the Human Body

The good news is that even though we may have subjected our bodies to years of acid abuse — abuse that is now manifesting itself in the form of increased infections and chronic tiredness — we still have the ability to reverse the effects of this abuse by restoring the body's pH balance to a healthy level. Everyone may learn to walk the tightrope of optimal health with enough practise; maintaining optimal health is a delicate balancing act.

As was discussed before, alcohol abuse may lead to a variety of health-related issues. When a critical amount of acid enters our system, it may damage our cells and organs if the acid is not neutralised in an appropriate manner.

To avoid this, one must ensure that the pH level is kept in a stable and stable balance. It is not difficult to determine whether or not our bodies have a higher level of alkaline by doing a simple test. This may be accomplished with the use of pH strips, which can be purchased at any pharmacy. There are two different kinds of "trp," one of which is used for the saliva, and the other is used for the pee.

In most cases, the amount of acid that your body produces may be determined by the pH level of your saliva; the normal range for this value is somewhere between 6.5 and 7.5 during the course of the day. A test to determine the urine's pH level will show the amount of acid in the urine; a normal value should be between 6.0 and 6.5 in the morning, and between 6.5 and 7.0 in the evening.

Accuracy at a Very High Level Is Toxic to the Physical System

These symptoms point to a high amount of acid in the body. If you suffer from chronic weariness, headaches, and frequent bouts of the common cold and flu, you may have too much acid in your body. The impact of acid on the body not only prevents the common illnesses that we are familiar with, but it also prevents other diseases from which you may suffer if your body has an excessive amount of acid.

The excessive amount of acidity in our bodies has been linked to a number of negative health effects, including depression, ulcers, dry skin, acne, and obesity, to name a few. Not limited to these, but also include other critical and potentially fatal disorders such as osteoporosis, bronchitis, respiratory infections, and cardiovascular conditions.

Because the cause of the problem has not been eliminated entirely, the symptoms may persist even if you take medicine to treat them, but this does not mean that your health will improve. Taking more medication will simply make the problem worse.

How To Perform A Water Test Using Ph Strips

The pH level of the body is an important factor that plays a role in an individual's overall health. The pH of the body is affected by everything, including the food we eat, the beverages we drink, and even our vitamin intake.

Even while it is ideal for the body to keep its pH level in the range of 7.35 to 7.45, it is not abnormal for it to reach values that are somewhat higher. Utilising the pH test strips assists in maintaining an accurate record of the pH level inside your body.

There are three different biological fluids that may be used to determine the pH level of your body: saliva, urine, and any other bodily fluid. The procedure is straightforward. Insert the litmus paper strip as directed, and then watch for it to change colours. The findings are sent to you in a matter of a few minutes at most.

A chart with color-coded readings is given for free with the purchase of pH test strips. Determine the pH level of your body by comparing the colour of the test strip to the corresponding colour chart. Due to the naturally acidic nature of urine, it is not unusual to receive a value as low as 6.

Consuming food up to two hours before testing the pH of your saliva may provide inaccurate findings, despite the fact that the level of pH in the urine is the most reliable indicator. Those who are concerned that their blood alcohol level is either too high or too low should retest after two hours have passed.

The energy level of the body is impacted by the pH level of the body. A pH level that is out of equilibrium may cause symptoms such as weariness, a weakened immune system, poor breath, and disease.

Both a steady pH level and weight reduction may be contributed to by maintaining a healthy diet along with an active lifestyle. Consuming a diet that is rich in fruits and vegetables may assist the body in naturally maintaining an alkaline balance inside the body.

The Relationship Between Acidic Foods and Cancer Those who advocate for alkaline diets and those who sell alkaline water are of the opinion that excessively acidic diets lead the body to become too acidic, which in turn raises the risk of developing cancer. Although it is a fact that the immediate environment surrounding cancer cells may be acidic, you should be aware that this is because of differences in the way tumours create energy and utilise oxygen in comparison to healthy tissues, and not because of the acidic foods (such as meats, dairy products, and eggs) that you consume.

In a similar vein, realise that their solution, which involves increasing your consumption of healthier alkaline foods such as vegetables, fruits, and alkaline water, will not in any way alter the pH level of your body. There are a variety of reasons why vegetables are beneficial to your health. reason: they contain a large amount of anti-inflammatory and cancer-preventing nutrients such as vitamins, minerals, and antioxidants. These nutrients are found in abundance in these foods.

People who drink alkaline water report overall health improvements, which may be ascribed to the simple fact that they are drinking more water, which results in improved hydration and detoxification. Alkaline water is beneficial for both of these purposes. There is also something known as the placebo effect.

In addition, alkaline water may include a greater mineral concentration, which is known to have beneficial effects on one's health, especially when one's diet consists mostly of processed or junk food, both of which are relatively poor in nutrients. This is especially important in cases when one's diet is deficient in nutrients.

pH-Level of Alkalinity

The word pH is an abbreviation for the "potential" of "Hydrogen." It refers to the total number of hydrogen ions that are present in a particular solution. The higher the concentration of on, the more acidic the oluton. The oluton will be more alkaline (base) if there are less on in it. pH is measured on a scale that goes from 0 to 14, with 7 being considered neutral on this scale. If the pH number is lower, then the substance is more acidic, and if the number is higher, then the substance is more alkaline. For instance, a pH level of 3 has a higher acidic concentration than a pH level of 5, but a pH level of 9 has a higher alkaline concentration than a pH level of 6. Consuming alkaline ionised water on a daily basis will assist in restoring a healthy balance as well as raising the body's ph level.

When it comes to humans, an alkaline pH level is considered normal for all tissues and fluids of the body (with the exception of the stomach). The pH level that is most important in the blood. In order to keep the blood at a precise pH between 7.35 and 7.45 (slightly alkaline), all of the other organs and fluids in the body will experience fluctuations within their range. The procedure is referred to as homeostasis. The human body is constantly adjusting the pH of its tissues and fluids in order to maintain a very narrow pH range in the blood. This is done so that the body can function properly.

D'etestprobablement la modification la plus importante. A person should try to limit the amount of meat, alcoholic beverages, soft drinks, caffeine, coffee, most nuts, eggs, vinegar, sauerkraut, ascorbic acid, cheese, white sugar, and medicinal drugs that they consume on a regular basis. Your diet should include more ripe fruits, vegetables, bean sprouts, water, milk, onions, figs, carrots, and beets, as well as more mo.

Testing the pH Level The pH level of the body may most accurately be determined by testing the pH of the saliva. Wait two hours after eating before doing the tet 'alva ritual. Into a spoon you should spit. Take a dip in the trp. Read it as soon as possible. Make use of the colour chart that corresponds to the right signal. A reading of 7.5 is considered to be optimal. This identifies a body that is just slightly alkaline.

In order to test urine: First thing in the morning, you should have a urine sample tested. A little cup should be filled with urine, and then a drop should be made into the cup. Read it as soon as possible. Results: 7.0, which is considered impartial. A value of 6.5 is considered to be rather acidic. A value of less than 6.5 is considered to be extremely acdc. Note: A reading of 8.0 or above, although not uncommon, suggests that the body has an excessive amount of alkalinity. Urine has a somewhat higher acid content than saliva does. [fromPhion, Inc., the company that produces pH trp]

Concerning the Regulation of the pH Individuals who have painful deposits anywhere on their feet can have a pH of

4.5 in their morning urine. At this hour (4.5), it is probably safe to assume that a significant amount of precipitation has fallen again throughout the night. Your body's pH may fluctuate during the day. This is completely normal. The process through which the urine becomes more alkaline after a meal is referred to as the "alkaline tide." If you ate three meals every day, you would get three alkaline tides. You will have the opportunity to dissolve some of your foot deposit throughout these periods, which last for about an hour each. These periods occur at regular intervals. However, if you let your pH drop to an unsafe level throughout the night, you will have to add the buffer back in. The overall effect will determine whether or not your savings increase or decrease.

Items that have traditionally been used to assist nutritionally in maintaining a normal pH level inside the body. The usage of these things is a traditional practise, and they are not intended to be prescribed for, to treat, or to claim that they may cure any disease, including cancer. disease associated with either a high or low pH level. Choose one of the following options to help alkalize your body before going to bed:

Take calcium (pure calcium carbonate or coral calcium) in an amount equivalent to 750 mg, and then add magnesium oxide in an amount equal to 300 mg. Calcium is easier to dissolve and maintain in a solution with the assistance of magnesium. It is not a good idea to take a large amount of calcium all at once since it cannot be digested or absorbed in any case, and doing so might make you constipated. Only one calcium pill per day is recommended for elderly patients. To assist in the dissolving process, take calcium tablets together with vitamin C or lemon water (1/4 teaspoon of vitamin C powder; adding honey is OK).

One tablet of magnesium oxide, dissolved in one cup of thermally processed milk or buttermilk, which may be either warm or cold.

(theaddition of cinnamon works just well). If these two treatments are successful for you, the pH of your morning urine will rise to 6.0; but, if for some reason they are not successful, you may need to take more extreme measures. Consume the nutritional supplements and milk earlier in the day, and save your sleep time for the following:

You should take some Balanced Bicarb Antacid, which is prepared by mixing three parts baking soda with one part potassium bicarbonate. It's possible that this potion might help with occasional allergic responses as well. At bedtime, take one level teaspoon in a glass of water. If your pH is 6 when you wake up, you should keep taking this amount every night until it drops below 6. If it does not, then take one and a half teaspoons. Keep an eye on your pH level since it will gradually return to normal, at which point you will need less and less acid.

This is a short list of alkaline foods that may help maintain a healthy pH balance:

pH of lemons and watermelons is 9.0

pH levels of 8.5 are found in bell pepper, kelp, mango, melon, parley, papaya, and seaweeds.

Peas, avocados, apples, pears, grapes, fruit juice, apricots, grape juice, and fruit juice all have a pH of 8.0.

Mushrooms, onions, almonds, egg yolks, tofu, soy milk, vinegar, tomatoes, cucumbers, coconut, and brown rice are the ingredients that go into this dish. - pH 7.5

A few common things, including the following, are known to leave an acidic ash in the bloodstream:

Most municipal water has a pH of 7.0.

pH level of distilled water is 6.5

6.0 on the pH scale for distilled water, fruit juice with added sugar, cigarettes, tobacco, and wine

White rice, ground beef, white flour, sugar, and sweetened yoghurt all have a pH of 5.5.

pH of acid:

Reverend OmololuAdeboye White bread, coffee, and water all have a pH of 4.0.

The pH of cola, soft drinks, beer, and hard liquor is 3.0.

pH 1.0 for an acd battery used in a car

Behaviours and feelings that produce acid include:

Overwork, anger, fear, jealousy, physical stress, and emotional stress all contribute to stress. You may alkalize your body by consuming alkaline foods and drinking alkaline water.

Stick to meals high in alkalinity while minimising your consumption of foods high in acidity.

Eat a lot of green and red foods.

Every day, you should consume at least 1.5 litres of alkaline water.

Aerobic activities, yoga, tai chi, walking, swimming, rebounding, and having a positive mind all contribute to an alkaline environment in the body.

Maintain the body in the best possible condition of health:

1) An acid-alkaline balance, also known as a pH balance or a Yin-Yang balance in terms of traditional Chinese medicine, is essential to achieving and maintaining one's best possible state of health. It is not a coincidence that yogis, Taoist masters, and Qigong masters all lead lives that are harmonious, alkaline, and balanced. Acne, imbalance, and physical weakness brought on by a poor diet and excessive use of alcohol, tobacco, and other drugs, as well as exposure to hazardous environmental factors, are very prevalent in the majority of Americans.

Drinking alkaline water is the complete and most effective way to neutralise free radicals, acdc waste, and carcnogen, and to flush out the accumulated toxins, all of which are electron-loving, and it provides the best hydration to each cell in the body. Microstructure, electron-rich, reducing alkaline water is the smallest antioxidant in molecular size.

Dessert Made With Chia Seeds And Almonds

Ingredients:

- 1 tbsp. maple syrup
- ⅓ fresh strawberries, hulled and sliced
- 2 tbsp. almonds, sliced
- 2 c. unsweetened almond milk
- ½ c. chia seeds
- 1 tsp. organic vanilla extract

Directions

Put the first four ingredients plus the extract into a large bowl and mix until everything is thoroughly combined.

Keep in the refrigerator for about three to four hours, stirring periodically.

To serve, top each portion with the cut strawberries and almond slices.

Advantages To Be Obtained From Adhering To An Alkaline Diet

The following is a list of the health advantages of the alkaline diet that have been verified by scientific research and which have also been reported by a significant number of people who follow the alkaline diet.

Improved health of the kidneys

The kidneys' ability to function properly is directly proportional to the degree of cleanliness of the blood. If there are a lot of toxins or other excretory products in the blood, the kidneys will have to work harder to cleanse the blood. This is because the blood contains both of these types of substances. renal injury or other blockages in renal function may be the result of an internal environment that is acidic, toxic, and saturated, as well as having a low pH.

Reduces the Odds of Developing Cancer

The alkaline diet is recommended by experts to sustain healthy body cells when chemotherapy is being administered because of their belief that alkaline foods may aid in the treatment of cancer. People who had cancer and were put on an alkaline diet exhibited strong signs of improvement, despite the fact that there is no established medical proof or research that have been undertaken that might clearly relate the strategy to the treatment of cancer.

impact that is anti-aging

There is currently no substance that has been identified that can totally reverse the ageing process; however, there are a number of strategies that can be used to slow down the process of ageing. One of them is following an alkaline diet, although despite its name, it is not a "Fountain of Youth." Therefore, you shouldn't have any expectations of miracles, since this won't add any more years to your life. Because its benefits may be seen on the skin, nails, and hair, it not only makes you feel younger but also helps you appear younger and feel better overall. Your nails will get stronger, your hair will become more shiny, and your skin will recover its brightness and flexibility.

Protects Against the Osteoporosis

The disorder known as osteoporosis is characterised by a weakening of the bones, which may occur either as a result of an insufficient amount of calcium being absorbed by the body or as a result of calcium being lost from the bones. Under these circumstances, the calcium will be expelled from the body through the urine. The alkaline diet has been shown in certain situations to be helpful in lowering the amount of calcium that is lost from the body. As a result, the bones are able to keep their resilience and structure. The individual's bones will naturally develop and fix themselves as he increases the amount of vegetables and fruits in his diet while decreasing the amount of processed food he consumes. Although the diet cannot stop the illness from occurring entirely, it may assist in keeping the condition under control.

Strong and Healthy Muscles

The muscles may lose their bulk, strength, and shape as we get older, which can lead to an increased risk of fractures and falls as we get older. The two most prominent side effects are pain and weakness.

enhanced vitality and physical strength

The alkaline diet maintains a consistent level of energy throughout the day by preventing any kind of sugar rush that may be brought on by the use of sweeteners, sugary foods, and carbonated beverages. If you put this life plan to the test, you will find that it is easier to exercise self-discipline since it forces you to decide when and what you will eat, which in turn will result in more restful sleeps. A cumulative impact of improved energy and vitality is produced as a result of all of these elements working together.

Helps your body get ready for its upcoming weight reduction.

This diet does not guarantee you will lose a significant amount of weight, but it may help your body get into the proper metabolic state to shed excess fat. The alkaline diet may be able to assist you in achieving your ideal body weight, often known as your Body Mass Index (BMI). This diet is not intended to help people lose weight; however, if you are overweight and have a slow metabolism, following this diet may help speed up your metabolism, which in turn may cause you to lose weight. You will also get rid of toxins, which will reduce the burden that the fat tissue is bearing and make it more readily accessible to be burnt off as energy. Additionally, the alkaline diet raises your energy levels, which might provide you with additional desire to engage in physical activity and further your weight loss efforts.

Reduced instances of constipation and bloating

An additional advantage of this diet, or remedy as some dietitians like to call it, is that it affects both your urine and faeces in a positive way. After following an alkaline diet for a short period of time, you will notice that your faeces are soft and that your urine is clear. This will happen as a result of your body operating correctly, which will result in more regular bowel motions for you.

Increased Prosperity

Within our bodies, hormones play the role of a catalyst for change and function. There is no way for any of the metabolic processes to be carried out without the production of some kind of hormone. The consumption of an alkaline diet contributes to an increase in the body's overall hormone synthesis, particularly that of growth hormones. Memory is improved as a result of the hormones' ability to make the brain work more effectively. Overall, a person has the impression that they are healthier and more vibrant. The consensus amongst nutritionists and other experts is that an alkaline diet creates inside the hormone-producing cells the optimal environment for the creation of growth hormones.

Stronger vitality

In order for the body to generate and utilise energy effectively, it is necessary for the cells to carry out their functions appropriately. The normal functioning of cellular functions and the production of energy are both hindered by acidity. The cells are able to perform better when the environment is more alkaline. There will be an increase in the production of energy, which will then be available to the other cells so that they may utilise it. This will cause an increase in overall levels of energy.

More robust immunity

When all of the body's cells are in good condition, the immune system is able to do its job more effectively. It is essential that the cells maintain their integrity. Maintaining cellular integrity helps prevent infections in the body's cells. Infectious agents will have a tough time penetrating the barrier and causing problems. When there is a low degree of acidity in the body's pH, it will be difficult for the cells to maintain their structures in their whole. This will make it easier for infections and poisons to enter the body, which will result in greater harm being done. The cells will thereafter be changed as a result of these diseases and poisons.

Blueberry Muesli Compliant With The Alkaline Diet

INGREDIENTS:

- 1/2 teaspoon salt
- 1 3/4 cup milk
- 1 large egg
- 1 1/2 tablespoon unsalted butter (melted)
- 1 tablespoon vanilla extract
- Lemon wedge
- 2 cups rolled oats
- 1 cup blueberries
- 1/2 cup sliced almonds
- 2/3 cups maple syrup
- 1 teaspoon baking powder
- 1 1/2 teaspoon ground cinnamon

INSTRUCTIONS:

- In a medium saucepan set over medium heat, combine a part of the blueberries with some of the maple syrup, and stir in a little amount of the lemon juice.

• Continue to cook the berries until they become pliable.

•Whisk together the milk, egg, butter, vanilla extract, and almond extract in a separate dish.

•In a separate dish, mix together the oats, half of the almonds, the remainder of the maple syrup, baking powder, cinnamon, and salt.

•Butter a square baking dish that is 8 inches on all sides and preheat the oven to 375 degrees Fahrenheit.

• For the first layer, arrange the blueberries that have been coated in maple syrup.

•Following that, layer with the oat mixture, and then pour milk over the top.

• Sprinkle the remaining unsweetened blueberries and almonds over the top.

•Bake for about forty minutes, or until the top part acquires a golden appearance.

•Take out of the oven, and let to cool.

•Slice it up and put it on the table.

Overeating

Food servings in the United States are often rather large. When we go out to restaurants, we have meals that are big enough for two people to share. This is in line with our expectations. We have been led to think that we need substantial portions of food due to our conditioning. This just is not the case.

I used to believe that more was better when it came to eating, but now I know that less really is more. Your health will improve if you eat less food. More life and energy.Additional vitality.More happiness.

When there is less food on your plate, you will be able to appreciate the flavours more fully. You are going to become more mindful of your eating and enjoy the food more. You will quickly discover that you have a greater sense of satisfaction. A greater sense of energy. You will discover that you are able to do more with less nourishment. Do more and achieve more. Learn more here. Experience more.

This is what takes place when a person makes a deliberate decision to eat healthily as opposed to subconsciously overeating. Your life will be different.

Even if you are consuming nutritious food, the unfavourable effects of overeating on a daily basis are still likely to occur. That much excess food is not essential, should not be wasted, and is not good for anyone's health. Consuming more than your body needs puts a burden on its organs and may cause your body to lose some of the alkalizing minerals that are stored in its cells, tissues, and bones. When you consume too much, you put your body in a nutritional state of imbalance, which may lead to inadequacies, toxic buildup, and blocked or sluggish lymphatic drainage.

When you were a young child, you had an innate awareness of when you were feeling hungry. You were able to gauge when you had eaten enough. We all have innate instincts, and if you pay attention to them, you'll discover that your body will continue to communicate with you about when it's time to eat and drink.

However, when you ingest stimulants and sugar, this causes a rise in your body's blood sugar level, which is subsequently followed by a fall in that level. This results in an increased need for sugar, which is necessary to rebalance the low blood sugar. Sometimes your body may advise you to eat even though you don't feel hungry at all. It has the sensation of hunger yet is not really hunger.

As soon as the stimulants in the diet are removed, the body's natural signals for when you are hungry and when you are full will begin to kick in again. You will then have an innate understanding of when to eat and when to stop eating. You won't need as much food to have the same satiated feeling. You will get an understanding of what is optimal for your own particular body in terms of quantity. When your body indicates that it needs food that will replenish it, you will eat a lot. When that is all that you need, you will find that you eat less.

It can be summed up like this. Consume food at the appropriate times. When you feel full, call it quits. And then, when you feel hunger setting in, eat once more. Savour every mouthful, take pleasure in each and every meal, and be content with the fact that you are supplying all of the cells in your body with healthy nourishment.

Performing an Analysis of Your pH Level

Whoever stated you needed to go to the doctor or a dietitian to get your pH checked was wrong. If someone has told you such, you should take into consideration the possibility that they are not very acquainted with the present world. It is important to know your pH level so that you can know where your body acid levels stand and also to get some insight on whether to eat acidic or alkaline foods. Testing for pH has become an activity that can be done with the snap of the finger and does not cause any complications or pain thanks to the pH testing kit that you can get from the store that is closest to you. It is also important to know that testing for pH has become a snap of the finger.

The litmus paper and a small pH chart are the two components that make up a pH test kit. You can perform a pH test on yourself by either contacting your saliva with one of the litmus paper pieces or contacting your urine with the paper. There is no complicated chemistry involved; the process is as simple as cutting a piece of cake. The following is an explanation of how to carry out each test.

When utilising one's own pee.

You may either pee directly on a section of the litmus paper or urinate into a container, after which you will dip the litmus paper; you will see a change in the colour of the litmus paper; after noticing this change, you will need to compare the colour of the litmus paper to the pH chart until it is comparable to the chart, and then determine whether the number is higher or lower than the chart. If your pH level is around seven, then everything is OK; however, if it dips below seven, this acts as an early warning to start an alkaline diet; it demonstrates that your body does not have the resources to maintain a desirable acid concentration.

If you want the greatest results while utilising saliva, it is recommended that you first rinse your mouth four times with clean water. Additionally, you should make sure that it has been more than two hours since you last brushed your teeth. After you have completed all of those steps, you have two options for testing: either spit directly into the litmus paper and watch for a change in colour, or spit into a container and then dip the litmus paper. Regardless of which option you choose, the outcome will be the same. After doing so, you can then compare the litmus paper to the pH chart and match its colour to the colour that is comparable to check the number on the top or bottom and if it's a seven, you're on the safe side, and if your pH level goes below seven, then it's time to start eating the alkaline diet properly.

Taking a few easy measures may help you attain a pH equilibrium.

Consume meals that are high in alkaline minerals to bring the pH level back into equilibrium.

It is not a tough effort to maintain a pH balance in the body; all that is required is the capacity to determine if a certain kind of food is acidic or alkaline, and then to be aware of what foods should be eaten in conjunction with it. For instance, earlier in the chapter there is an article about the best top ten alkaline foods, and there is also an article on the top ten foods to avoid because they are highly rich in acids. If a person is able to actually know whether they are eating an alkaline food or an acidic food, then they are able to substitute with corresponding, it's good to avoid eating pizza, but that doesn't necessarily mean cutting off from your favourite type of food, pizza is an acidifying fast food.

The same is true for consuming foods, vegetables, or drinks that are rich in extremely alkaline elements. Always be on the lookout for a complement; think of the situation as a game of "tit for tat."

Make room in your schedule for some R&R or plan a trip.

It is unhealthy to deny your body the opportunity to sleep; sleep is necessary for everyone, not just children; even machines are allowed time to cool down after they have been worked. To keep a good pH level relaxing the mind from all forms of stress and also sufficient sleep is necessary. People who rarely get time to sleep are most likely to be sick with high blood pressure or ulcers.

Stop using tobacco products and alcoholic beverages.

An alkaline diet leads to a longer life, and quitting smoking will definitely lead to a longer life. Smoking leads to a large intake of chemicals in the body, which triggers acid production in a desperate effect for the body to neutralise. A single cigarette contains over a thousand chemicals, all of which are harmful to health. Beer drinking may also produce a big imbalance in the pH level adversely; beer kills the liver and the pancreases, which are both the key components of the body responsible for balancing and creating acid.

Purification on both the inside and outside of the human body

The foods and vegetables that we put into our bodies may have an effect on the pH level, but so can the chemicals and other environmental variables that are present in the atmosphere. Because we live in a world where chemicals from factories and other industries fill the air, it is important for us to make sure that we always have some alkaline rich foods or vegetables with us wherever we go. It is also advisable to practise cleaning your homestead to eliminate any acid forming substance that might be inhalable. Both of these things should be done regularly.

The Process through Which the Digestive System Destroys Food

As food moves through the digestive system, the organs that line the path begin to break it down utilising motion and the fluids that they produce:

Movement include squeezing, chewing, and combining

Bile, stomach acid, and enzymes are examples of digestive juices.

Beginning with the moment when you put the meal into your mouth for the first time:

Salivation is formed in the mouth as a result of chewing, which takes place in the mouth. The digesting liquid that is found in saliva coats the food, making it more pliable and facilitating its passage down the oesophagus and into the stomach. In addition, saliva creates an enzyme that kickstarts the process of converting the carbohydrates in your diet into glucose.

Oesophagus: when you swallow, the peristaltic action transports the food into your stomach, and it does so by way of the oesophagus.

The digestive process begins in the stomach, where glands create enzymes and acid to help digest meals. Your meals and these liquids are mixed together by the muscles in your stomach.

Pancreas: This organ is responsible for producing digestive juice, which includes enzymes that are necessary for the breakdown of fatty tissue, protein, and carbohydrates. Ducts, which are similar to tiny tubes, are responsible for transporting the pancreatic juice to the small intestine.

The liver is responsible for the production of bile, which is another digestive liquid that assists in the breakdown of vitamins and fats. The bile will be transported through the bile ducts to either the gallbladder for storage or the small intestine to be used.

Gallbladder The gallbladder is a pear-shaped organ that sits under the liver and stores bile in between meals. After eating, bile travels via the bile ducts and into the small intestine, where it is needed for digestion.

The small intestine is where digestive juice is produced, where it is combined with bile and the juices produced by the pancreas, and where the last stages of the digestion of fat, carbohydrates, and proteins take place. The bacteria in your digestive tract create certain enzymes that assist in the digestion of carbohydrates, and water is drawn from your circulation to assist in the process of breaking down the food you eat. In addition, both water and nutrients are absorbed through the small intestine.

In the large intestine, more water is drawn in from the digestive system, and bacteria in the gut contribute to the process of breaking down what nutrients are still there in order to make vitamin K. The stool is formed from all of the waste materials.

Where the Food That Has Been Digested Goes

The majority of the nutrients that are obtained from the food you eat are absorbed by the small intestine, and the circulatory system subsequently transports these nutrients to various parts of the body, either for utilisation or for storage. The blood carries amino acids, simple sugars, glycerol, and certain minerals and vitamins to your liver, which will then digest them and store them for distribution to other areas of the body when they are required. There are specialised cells that help nutrients pass through the intestinal wall and into the circulation. These cells help the nutrients enter the bloodstream.

The lymph system is a network of vessels that circulates lymph fluid and white blood cells throughout your body to aid in the absorption of vitamins and fatty acids as well as the battle against infectious diseases. The body makes use of carbohydrates, fatty acids, amino acids, and glycerol in order to construct the components necessary for cellular repair, growth, and the production of energy.

What Determines the Outcome of the Digestive Process?

Signals go to and from your digestive system all the way up to your brain, as well as inside the digestive tract itself. This is a collaborative effort between your nerves and your hormones.

Your stomach and small intestine are coated with cells that create and release hormones that serve to manage the digestive system. These hormones are produced by the cells that line your stomach and small intestine. The hormones will indicate to the body when digestive juices are required and will also communicate with the brain about whether or not you are full. Important hormones for the gastrointestinal tract are also produced by the pancreas.

Nerves Your digestive system is connected to your central nervous system, which consists of your spinal cord and brain, and your nerves assist to regulate some of the processes of your digestive system. When you are exposed to the sight or scent of food, your brain will transmit signals that will cause your salivary glands to activate, causing your mouth to start watering.

There is also something called the Enteric Nervous System (ENS), which refers to the nerves that are found in the walls of the digestive system. When you eat, the walls of the gastrointestinal tract expand, and the nerves that control these muscles release a number of chemicals that either slow down or speed up the rate at which food travels through the system and causes the production of digestive juices. In addition, the nerves will transmit signals that govern the tightening and relaxing of the muscles in the gastrointestinal system.

Those who suffer from GERD or acid reflux are well aware that digestion doesn't always go according to plan, despite the fact that this is the way it is supposed to function.

How the buildup of acid in the body causes weakness

When the pH of the body's internal environment gets too acidic, there are three distinct ways in which illness might manifest inside the body:The first one has to do with the process that enzymes go through. Enzymes are the "labourer drones" that are responsible for each and every one of the biochemical changes that take place in the body as well. These changes are essential to the normal functioning of the organs. Enzymes are only able to carry out their tasks correctly in environments with a pH that has been carefully controlled; otherwise, their activity might become disrupted or possibly halt entirely. Illness manifests itself as soon as their activity level is even slightly reduced. In the case that there is a disruption, the body is now in a position where it cannot operate correctly, which ultimately leads to death. Before this terrible stage, a variety of diseases began to manifest as an increasing number of enzymes discovered that the interior environment had become more acidic, which flipped the enzymes' world upside down. -The second reason why the body becomes ill is because of the harsh and destructive nature of acids that are present in excess inside the tissues. This is the reason why the body gets sick. Acids irritate the organs that they come into touch with, which may ultimately lead to the death of the organisms by alkaline chemicals. Lesions or tissue that has been hardened as a consequence of inflammation may sometimes be exceedingly painful. This has a significant impact on organs like the skin and kidneys, whose primary function is to eliminate strong acids from the body. The disruption that is caused by abnormally acidic perspiration is responsible for a significant number of cases of dermatitis, hives, tingling, and red patches that appear on the skin. The most susceptible places are those that tend to accumulate perspiration, such as the armpits, the backs of the knees, beneath the diapers of newborns, and the band of a wristwatch. When the urine has an excessive amount of acid, it is very painful to urinate, and the urinary system "burns," becomes polluted (cystitis), or becomes inflamed (urethritis).

A scorching feeling in the anus, arthritis, neuritis, enteritis, and colitis are only some of the illnesses that may be brought on by strong acid. These illnesses are invisible to the naked eye but can be felt very clearly by the afflicted. Because of the acid's pervasive presence, the tissues are in a vulnerable state, which renders them defenceless against microbial or viral infection. For example, lesions of the mucous layers of the respiratory system make it easier for microorganisms to penetrate the tissues and replicate there. This is made worse by the fact that the viability of the immune system may also be inhibited by acid activity, which reduces the production and strength of white blood cells whose purpose it is to fight against microorganisms. - This makes the situation much worse. The loss of minerals is the third cause of having an excess of acid in the body. Since the body releases alkaline minerals to destroy acids, this causes the body to lose minerals. As a result of the fact that alkaline minerals are stored in each and every tissue of the body, this demineralization may have a very significant impact and can have an effect on any organ. The most common side effects of demineralization are problems that affect the bones and teeth. Bones lose their calcium, and along with it, their capacity to resist and adapt. As a result, bones become more brittle, lose their density, develop rheumatism, and erode the intervertebral disc, also known as (sciatica). The lack of minerals may also cause teeth to become more susceptible to damage over time. They are prone to chipping, becoming hypersensitive to hot and cold food, and increasing their vulnerability to holes. The fragility caused by demineralization causes hair to lose its lustre and vigour, and it also causes hair to begin falling out in an increased quantity. Even the tiniest influence causes the fingernails to split and break, the skin to dry up and crack or wrinkle, and the gums to bleed and become sensitive.

Questions That Have Been Asked Before, Section Seven

Since I was first made aware of The Alkaline Diet, I've had to do a significant amount of study on the subject. That is not a problem for me since I take pleasure in doing my own research, or at least I have trained myself to take pleasure in doing so. On the other hand, I have developed a list of a few questions that I am often asked in order to help those individuals who either don't have a lot of time or just aren't interested in obtaining knowledge.

Is there any truth to the alkaline diet?
Both yes and no. That is to say that it is effective provided that you adhere to it in the correct manner. I began this plan with the purpose of going into it half-assed, and the outcomes came out precisely the same way: half-assed. In the beginning, I started this plan with the idea of going into it half-assed. If shedding some pounds is your primary

objective, you should have realistic expectations. This diet is an excellent choice for anyone who, like myself, are trying to improve their general health in addition to their weight loss efforts. Altering the chemical make-up of your body is going to be the primary emphasis of this programme. In other words, you want to bring down the naturally occurring acidity and bring up the alkalinity. This will not only assist you in losing a few pounds, but it will also assist you in appearing and feeling years younger.

What kind of food can you eat?
This was the part of the process that required the least amount of investigation. Online, I searched for "Can Eat" lists, and the ones I discovered didn't seem to be very limiting in their recommendations. As was said earlier, the objective is to decrease the amount of natural acid that is produced by your body by increasing the consumption of foods that are high in alkaline. This include the vast majority of fruits and

vegetables, as well as soybeans and tofu. In addition to that, you might try eating some legumes, nuts, or seeds.

What foods are off limits for you?

And now, the list of those meals that you should avoid completely is presented before you. This is the same as any other strategy that encourages you to lead a healthy lifestyle that you could choose to follow. Foods that are high in protein should not be included in your diet at this time. This contains a variety of meats, dairy products, and eggs. Remove any processed items from your diet, such as snacks that are pre-packaged or canned. These are all examples of foods that are classified as acidic. Avoid drinking any drinks that include caffeine or alcohol. Because I enjoyed diet drinks so much, this was by far the toughest challenge for me. (I bet you thought I was going to mention something about drinking, didn't you?) It is possible to get past this obstacle. Drinking an alkaline beverage, such as green tea, prior to eating moderate quantities of alcohol or caffeine is recommended. This is something that you should only consider doing if you have made significant progress with the programme and have a good idea of the kinds of foods that won't bother you.

Is maintaining an alkaline diet a costly endeavour?
This is a very important issue to ask since, as you are well aware, there are a great number of plans that have monthly premiums that are more expensive than a typical mortgage payment. That is not the case in this instance. Because you are exchanging more costly junk food for fresh fruits and veggies that cost less money, you may even end up with some more money in your pocket. And here's a major one: by improving your health, you may be able to reduce the amount of money you spend on co-pays and medications at the doctor's office. that's funny to say that, yet it is in fact accurate. The cost of trips to the doctor may quickly build up for those who have inadequate or no health insurance.

Consider obtaining some nutritional supplements that might be of assistance to you in your endeavour if you don't mind spending a little more money. Even if you want to learn more about the diet, you don't have to buy any books in order to perform research on it. There is a wealth of free information available on the internet, which contains a big list of foods that are healthy and those that are unhealthy, as well as a list of dos and don'ts.

How can I learn to create meals that are better for me?
Cooking is something new for people like me who grew up eating fast food three times a day, seven days a week (yes, that was me, except on Sunday when my mom cooked), so this may seem like an odd question to some people. But for those people, like me, who grew up eating fast food, this is a legitimate inquiry. To begin, make sure you follow the shopping lists. After you have bought all of the ingredients

required to cook nutritious meals, look up some recipes on the internet. There is an abundance of information available on how to cook nutritious meals. If that doesn't satisfy your appetite, go on over to Amazon.com and browse through some of the cookbooks there. There are even some free options. It's more of a game of trial and error than anything else.

Is it possible for acid in the body to alter one's mood?

Without a doubt! Acidic bodies and an overgrowth of microorganisms may ultimately lead to proportions that are out of control, which can result in a variety of mental health issues, including depression and other mood disorders. Studies have revealed that anxiety, panic attacks, irritability, and PMS are some of the additional adverse effects of acid in the body. These symptoms may get even more severe as acid levels grow in the body. (You are aware, ladies, that this is the very last thing we need.)

Does weariness result from acid exposure?

Yes, having high amounts of acid is one of the numerous variables that might produce weariness, but there are many more as well. In point of fact, weariness is most likely the most prominent sign or complaint of having a body that is too acidic. To take this a step further, some studies suggest that allergies and sinus infections, both of which I have had in the past, are also one of the negative effects of this medication. Just so you know, ever since I started following this diet, I've had less episodes of sinusitis and allergy flare-ups.

What Are The Pros And Cons Of Following An Alkaline Diet?

Added Benefits

This dietary pattern, which is distinguished by its emphasis on fresh produce, does not need for an excessive amount of time spent preparing meals or an advanced level of culinary expertise. Eat more fruits and veggies, along with some grains and natural oils, and you should be good to go. However, there is no evidence from scientific research to support claims that an alkaline diet may be beneficial for weight loss and the prevention of sickness. On the other hand, there is some evidence to suggest that some aspects of the diet could really be good for one's health.

Helps to Preserve Muscle Mass: You may be able to keep more lean muscle mass as you become older by following an alkaline diet. In a clinical trial that took place over the course of three years and included 384 men and women over the age of 65, researchers revealed that a high intake of potassium-rich foods, such as fruits and vegetables in an alkaline diet, may enable older adults to preserve their muscular power as they age.

A possibility Contribute to the Avoidance of Diabetes: It's possible that diabetes may be avoided by eating foods that aren't acidic. In a study that was published in Diabetologia, the researchers looked at 66,485 different women over the course of 14 years. During that time span, medical professionals identified 1,372 people who had not previously been diagnosed with diabetes. In a study where the participants' eating habits were analysed, researchers found that women whose diets included the greatest levels of alkaline foods had a significantly elevated risk of developing diabetes. The authors of the research suggest that a high intake of foods rich in acidity may be associated to insulin resistance.

Contradictions in terms

Consuming certain foods that have the ability to alter the body's ph level may, according to the alkaline diet, lead to improvements in one's health. However, there is no evidence from scientific research to show that following a diet low in acid confers any significant benefits. Listed below are some drawbacks to the strategy for the diet.

Inadequate Supply of Dairy Products: On a diet that excludes dairy products, it may be more difficult to get enough of some essential minerals, such as calcium, magnesium, phosphorous, and potassium. These minerals may be found in milk products. According to dietary specialists, removing dairy products from one's diet makes it almost impossible to get the recommended daily amount of calcium, which is important for maintaining healthy bones. In addition, consuming just vegetables might be challenging when trying to meet calcium needs. Even while certain plants, like spinach, have a high amount of oxalates and phytic acid, which are known to bind calcium, very little of this calcium is actually absorbed by the body.

Insufficiency in Protein: Because the alkaline diet discourages the use of high-quality, bioavailable protein sources, it might be difficult to consume the required amount of protein while adhering to the alkaline diet. According to the standards that are now in place, an adult's daily calorie intake should consist of anything from 10–35 percent protein. 8 Even while small amounts of protein may be found in fruits and vegetables, it is difficult to consume enough of either to meet one's daily requirements. A lack of protein may contribute to a range of health issues, including a reduction in muscle mass and compromised nutrition.

www.ingramcontent.com/pod-product-compliance
Lightning Source LLC
Chambersburg PA
CBHW051734020426
42333CB00014B/1301